1

TABLE OF CONTENTS

Overview of The Weight Watchers Freestyle Program

Weight Watchers work via a point system. The thing is that every food item is assigned a specified number of points called SmartPoints. When you follow Weight Watchers, you are only allowed a certain number of points daily thus helping you to portion out your food as well as consume those that have lesser point value to get the most out of the program.

Recently, Weight Watchers rolled on a new program that will definitely make you excited. Called the Weight Watchers Freestyle, it changes the Weight Watchers game. Under the new WW Freestyle program, more than 200 types of foods have been assigned with a SmartPoints value equal to Zero regardless of their calorie, sugar, protein, and saturated fat content. Thus said, people can eat without limit from the Zero Points food list.

What Will Change

There are a few changes that will happen under the WW Freestyle Program. So aside from the types of foods that will get new zero points, below are the big changes that have been implemented for this new Weight Watchers program.

- **Daily SmartPoints allowance will change:** In order to balance the new zero points food that are introduced, the daily SmartPoints allowance will be recalculated still according to your height, weight, age, and gender. So for instance, if you have been given 30 daily points in the previous plan, the new Freestyle SmartPoints will be smaller at 23.

- **New rollover points:** One of the newest features of the WW Freestyle Program is that you can roll over up to four unused daily points into your weekly points so that you can use it whenever you like for the rest of the week. This is really convenient especially if you are going to attend a big dinner on Saturday. You can start saving points during weekdays so that you can have more point allowance for that special day.

What Will Remain

Although a newer version of the Weight Watchers, the WW Freestyle Program has retained some of the old features of the original program. Below are the features the both Weight Watchers and WW Freestyle Program have in common:

- **SmartPoint:** The SmartPoint is the core of the Weight Watchers program. The WW Freestyle Program still utilizes the SmartPoints using the same calculation thus most of the foods (except for those with the new zero point items assigned to them) will have the same SmartPoint. Remember that the calculation of SmartPoints is based on saturated fat, calories, sugar, and protein. Foods that are high in saturated fat and sugar have higher SmartPoint values while those that are high in protein have lower SmartPoint value.

- **Weekly points allowance:** While the new WW Freestyle Program's daily point allowance will be recalculated to make room for the foods with new zero points, your weekly points allowance will remain the same.

- **Physical activity:** Physical activity will remain in the program. In fact, this program encourages you to be physically active. The amount of physical activity that you do will also depend on the points system of Weight Watchers.

- **Tracking:** You still need to track your weight on the Weight Watchers freestyle plan, but you only have to do that on foods that are not on the zero points list.

New Weight Watchers Freestyle Zero Smartpoints Food List

With the development of the Weight Watchers Freestyle Program, there are now many food items that are assigned with zero points. With this new SmartPoint assignment, these foods no longer need to be tracked or measured thus making it easier for many people to follow the program. Below are the types of foods that have been assigned with zero SmartPoints. It is important to take note that those that are not included in this list still retain their SmartPoint value.

Fruits

It is not much of surprise to find fruits in the zero list. After all, they were in the zero list in the previous plan. All fruits–fresh, frozen, or canned–are assigned with zero SmartPoint as long as they do not come with added sugar or are sugar-free. So if you are wondering if apples, bananas, grapes, strawberries, and blueberries have zero points, the answer is yes. What about very sweet fruits like dates and figs? Yes, they both come with zero points.

But while most fruits come with the zero SmartPoints, there are some fruits that are not included in the list. For instance, Avocados and plantains (cooking bananas) are not included in the WW Freestyle zero points list so make sure that you heed this warning.

On the other hand, smoothies should also need to be calculated for their SmartPoints even if they are made entirely out of fresh fruits and vegetables. The reason being is that when taken in liquid form, you have the tendency to consume more of fruits without the feeling of being full. Thus, you need to track the points.

Vegetables

Starchy vegetables such as sweet corn and peas, under the conventional Weight Watchers Program, are assigned with 1 SmartPoint. With the new WW Freestyle Program, some starchy foods have made it to the zero list.

Vegetables that are fresh, frozen or canned as long as they do not come with oil and are sugar-free come with zero points. So, eat as many cucumber, eggplant, daikon, pumpkin, sweet peppers, and radishes as they come with zero points.

While there are many vegetables that have made the zero list, there are some that did not make it to the cut. These include dried vegetables as they are considered more of a snack thus there is a tendency for people to overeat them. Potatoes and sweet potatoes did not make it to the list because of their high starch content as well as the fact that it is easy to over-consume them as a snack.

Beans

Beans and lentils of all sorts are considered as starchy vegetables. In the conventional Weight Watchers program, ½ cup of servings of beans is assigned with 3 SmartPoints. In the WW Freestyle Program, beans such as black beans, edamame, kidney, pinto, fava, lima, and soybeans are now assigned with zero points. Even lentils and bean sprouts are assigned with zero points.

Meats

Many followers of the new WW Freestyle Program are now rejoicing the fact that certain types of meats are now included in the zero list. In fact, never before has this program included any meats on their zero point list. But it is important to take note that not all meats are included in the zero list and only the skinless chicken and turkey made it into the list. Nevertheless, this is good news for many people.

A 3-ounce portion of chicken breasts without skin is assigned with 2 SmartPoints under the conventional Weight Watchers Program. With the new Freestyle Program, fat-free and skin-free chicken breasts, as well as chicken tenderloin (as long as skinless), is now assigned with zero points.

Similar with chicken, a serving of 3-ounce skinless turkey breast is assigned 3 SmartPoints. The new WW Freestyle Program assigns zero points to skinless turkey breast products such as ground turkey as well as turkey meat.

The thing is that not all lean meats have made it into the Freestyle zero list and these include lean pork and beef. The thing is that healthy diets recommend limiting the amount of the consumption of red meats. On the other hand, dried meats like turkey or chicken jerky are not included in the list as they are considered as snack foods and they can be overeaten by many.

Tofu

The Weight Watchers assign a serving of 3-ounces of tofu with 1 SmartPoint. The introduction of the new WW Freestyle Program awards the tofu with a new SmartPoint value equivalent to zero.

Eggs

Eggs are protein-rich foods that are assigned with a particular SmartPoint value on the conventional Weight Watchers Program. Under the old program, one egg is equivalent to 2 SmartPoints while 3 egg whites or ½ cup of egg substitute is equivalent to 1 SmartPoint. With the new program, both eggs and egg whites are no longer assigned with SmartPoints.

Non-fat Plain Yogurt

Getting more dairy into your diet can help you lose fat while preserving muscles at the same time. The Weight Watchers Program encourages you to incorporate milk into your diet. A cup of non-fat milk is equivalent to 3 SmartPoints. Yogurt, on the other hand, is a good source of protein and calcium and it also comes with 3 points per cup for the Greek non-fat type while 5 points per cup for regular non-fat yogurt.

The new WW Freestyle Program removed the assigned SmartPoint value on non-fat and sugar-free yogurt. These include traditional, Greek, Icelandic, as well as soy yogurt. Other dairy products like whole milk, non-fat milk, and cheese still retain their SmartPoint value.

Fish and Shellfish

Fish and shellfish are great sources of lean proteins. In the conventional Weight Watchers program, a 3-ounce portion of fish is equivalent to 3 points while tuna, tilapia, shrimps, and lobsters come with 1 point each. Fishes that are packed with Omega-3s like salmon and herring have 4 points per 3-ounce serving.

The new WW Freestyle program assigns all fish and shellfish—whether fresh, frozen, or canned – with zero SmartPoints as long as they are skinless and does not come with added oil and sugar. The types of fishes that have been identified good for the new WW Freestyle program include butterfish, carp, arctic char, anchovies, perch, pike, halibut, herring, mackerel, tuna, swordfish, tilapia, snapper, sardines, sea bass, roe, pompano, trout, salmon, and even all types of smoked fishes.

Tips to Succeed on The Weight Watchers Freestyle Program

If you are planning to attempt this new WW Freestyle program, there are several things that you need to do in order to succeed with this new program. Below are the top tips on how you can be successful in achieving your goals while following this particular weight loss program.

- **Incorporate as many zero points food as you can:** Learning the zero list by heart is very important because it will help you plan the types of foods that you should eat. When preparing meals and getting the most benefit out of the program, make sure that you include as many zero points food in your meals as possible but keep in mind that you need to plan carefully. Just because eggs are in the zero list does not mean that you have the freedom to eat 10 eggs in one sitting.

- **Drink plenty of water:** Drinking water is good for you and it can help you in your weight loss journey. It can also help you fight fatigue as well as improve your digestion. Moreover, water is practically calorie-free, so you can guzzle as much as you want without gaining any weight.

- **Plan your meals:** Just because you don't need to keep track of the food in the zero list, does not mean that you should not plan your meals. Meal planning may sound very difficult, but it can be an effective way to achieve your goals. This also makes meal preparation more fun.

- **Get active:** Physical exercise will help you achieve your fitness goals faster. In fact, the WW Freestyle program encourages you to exercise daily. If not, make sure that you exercise at least 3 times a week.

- **Bank your points for one delicious weekly treat:** The best thing about the WW Freestyle Program is that, while it gives you the understanding of how eating treats can affect your overall diet, it does not totally cut out sweets from your life. You can bank your daily point allowance and save them so that you can enjoy a delicious treat during the weekend. That way, you will be motivated to follow the program because you have something to look forward to during the weekend.

- **Make smart swaps for cravings:** Cravings while following the program is normal. This is especially true if you have been dieting for a few days. If it is hard to give in to your cravings, make smart swaps. For instance, if you have a sugar craving, try munching on a piece of fruit instead.

Weight Watchers Freestyle Program FAQs

Why are lean red meats with the same nutritional value as zero points meat like chicken breast not included in the list?

The US Department of Agriculture suggests limits of the consumption of red meats like pork, lamb, and beef as overconsumption may lead to health issues in the future. Even the American Heart Association and the American Institute for Cancer Research agree!

Is this program good for vegans and vegetarians?

This program is great for vegetarians and vegans as there are so many non-animal food items that are included in the zero point list. They have a wide variety of foods to choose from. They can benefit from the WW Freestyle Program.

Is the WW Freestyle Program similar to the Paleo Diet?

Remember that the Paleo Diet is a restrictive diet that does not allow you to eat dairy and grains. The WW Freestyle Program does not restrict you from eating any types of food groups.

What portion sizes should we eat when it comes to the zero points foods?

Good question. However, there is no set portion size or limits on the zero points food. These foods were chosen because they are less likely to be eaten. The aim here is for you to be satisfied but not stuffed so eat only what you can finish.

Will the dried version of the zero points food also be zero?

Dried pineapples often contain more calories than fresh pineapples of the same portion size, amount, or weight. The program promotes eating vegetables in their raw or cooked form. We consider dried vegetables and fruits as snack foods that can easily be overeaten. So, no. They don't meet the criteria of the zero points food.

Which plant-based products not included in the zero points list?

While tofu is considered as zero points food, tempeh and seitan are not included because they contain Ingredients: such as wheat and brown rice that, in essence, amount to specific SmartPoint values.

Are the SmartPoints for grocery and restaurant foods adjusted?

Yes. The Weight Watchers company has already updated the food database with the new zero points food. So, if you go to a restaurant or grocery store that serve or sell Weight Watchers products, the point system has already been adjusted for the WW Freestyle Program.

WEIGHT WATCHERS FREESTYLE PROGRAM BREAKFAST RECIPES

ZERO FSP BREAKFAST PANCAKES

Servings Per Recipe: 4

FSP: 0

Cooking Time: 5 minutes

Ingredients:

- ¼ tsp cinnamon
- 1 tsp vanilla
- 1 tsp baking powder
- 1 banana, mashed well
- 2 egg whites

Directions:

1. Place a griddle on medium fire and heat for at least 3 minutes.
2. In a medium bowl, whisk well egg whites.
3. Stir in cinnamon, vanilla, and baking powder.
4. Add mashed banana and mix thoroughly.
5. Evenly divide batter into 4 and cook for 2 minutes, flip and cook for half a minute. Repeat process for remaining batter.
6. Serve and enjoy with fresh berries.

ANOTHER EGG MUFFIN WITH 0 FSP

Servings Per Recipe: 12
FSP: 0
Cooking Time: 40 minutes

Ingredients:
- ¼ tsp marjoram
- ¼ tsp red pepper flakes
- ½ tsp black pepper
- ½ tsp salt
- ½ tsp sage
- ½-lb 99% fat-free ground turkey breast
- 1 green bell pepper, diced
- 1 tsp Montreal Steak seasoning blend
- 12 eggs

Directions:
1. Place a nonstick skillet on medium-high fire and lightly grease with cooking spray.
2. Preheat oven to 350°F and lightly grease muffin tins with cooking spray.
3. Add ground turkey on skillet and sauté. Season with marjoram, red pepper flakes, black pepper, salt, and sage. Mix well and cook for 8 minutes or until no longer pink.
4. Meanwhile, in a bowl, whisk well the eggs and season with steak seasoning blend and stir in diced bell pepper. Combine thoroughly.
5. Once ground turkey is done cooking, evenly divide into the 12 muffin tins.
6. Pour egg mixture on top of ground turkey.
7. Pop in the oven and for 30 minutes bake.
8. Serve and enjoy.

SALSA ROASTED SALMON

Servings Per Recipe: 2

FSP: 0

Cooking Time: 15 minutes

Ingredients:
- 1 plum tomato, chopped
- ½ small onion, chopped
- 1 clove of garlic, minced
- Small jalapeno pepper, chopped
- 1 tsp apple cider vinegar
- ½ tsp chili powder
- ¼ tsp ground cumin
- ¼ tsp salt
- 3 dashes of Tabasco hot sauce
- 2 4-ounce salmon fillets

Directions:
1. Preheat the oven to 400°F.
2. In a food processor, mix the all the Ingredients: except for the salmon fillets. Blend until well combined.
3. Place the salmon in a roasting pan and pour the salsa on top.
4. Place inside the oven and roast for 15 minutes or until the salmon gets flaky.

SCRAMBLED EGGS WITH SPINACH

Servings Per Recipe: 6

FSP: 1

Cooking Time: 10 minutes

Ingredients:

- 1 ½ tbsps extra virgin olive oil
- ½ cup 2% sharp cheddar cheese
- 1 tsp salt
- 1 tsp pepper
- 1 clove garlic, crushed and minced
- ½ red onion, diced
- 3 cups organic baby spinach
- 1 organic tomato, diced
- 6 large eggs

Directions:

1. Whisk well salt, pepper, and eggs in a large bowl.
2. Place a large nonstick skillet on medium high fire and add oil. Heat for a minute.
3. Sauté garlic and onions for 5 minutes. Stir in tomatoes and sauté for 3 minutes.
4. Stir in spinach and cook for 2 minutes or until starting to wilt.
5. Pour in eggs and cook for 5 minutes, occasionally stirring.
6. Serve and enjoy.

No-Cook Oats and Peanut Butter

Servings Per Recipe: 1
FSP: 7
Prep Time: 5 minutes

Ingredients:
- 1 tbsp sugar free jam
- 1 tbsp peanut butter
- ¾ cup almond milk
- ½ cup old-fashioned oats

Directions:
1. In a bowl with lid, mix all Ingredients: except for the jam.
2. Cover and set in the fridge overnight.
3. Enjoy with a tablespoon of jam.

EASY AND DELICIOUS BREAKFAST CASSEROLE

Servings Per Recipe: 6

FSP: 5

Cooking Time: 50 minutes

Ingredients:
- 1 cup light grated cheese, divided
- ¾ cup diced onion
- 1 cup diced peppers
- 8-oz diced cooked ham
- 1 cup skim milk
- 3 egg whites
- 5 eggs
- 1 7.5-oz package Pillsbury biscuits

Directions:
1. Preheat oven to 350°F and grease a 9x13-inch casserole dish.
2. Spread Pillsbury biscuits evenly on bottom of dish.
3. In a large bowl, whisk well eggs and egg whites.
4. Pour in milk and mix well.
5. Add onion, peppers, ham, and 2/3 cup of cheese. Whisk to combine and pour on top of biscuits.
6. Cover dish with foil and bake for 30 minutes.
7. Uncover and spread cheese on top and bake uncovered for another 15-20 minutes or until top is set and cheese is starting to brown.
8. Serve and enjoy while hot.

HAM AND EGG BREAKFAST SANDWICH

Servings Per Recipe: 2

FSP: 5

Cooking Time: 10 minutes

Ingredients:

- 4 tbsps shredded asiago cheese, divided
- 4-oz deli ham
- 1 tbsp ranch dressing
- A dash of paprika
- Pepper and salt to taste
- 1 tbsp milk
- 1 egg white
- 1 egg
- 2 everything flat-out fold it bread

Directions:

1. Pick a bowl that can fit your bread in and whisk well paprika, pepper, salt, milk, egg white, and eggs.
2. Place a medium nonstick frypan on medium fire and let it heat.
3. Meanwhile, spread dressing over each fold and add 2 tbsps of cheese and 2-oz of ham on each bread.
4. Dip bread in bowl of egg, thoroughly and place in pan.
5. Cook for 5 minutes and turnover and cook for another 5 minutes.
6. Serve and enjoy.

Egg and Ham Muffins

Servings Per Recipe: 12
FSP: 3
Cooking Time: 20 minutes

Ingredients:
- Paprika, pepper, and salt to taste
- 12 eggs
- 12 slices of ham, no preservatives

Directions:
1. Preheat oven to 375°F.
2. With ham, line muffin tin with 1 ham each.
3. Break the eggs one at a time with one egg introduced inside the cupped ham.
4. Season each muffin with pepper, salt, and paprika to taste.
5. Pop in the oven and bake for 20 minutes.
6. Once done, serve and enjoy.

Bacon and Zucchini Egg-Muffin

Servings Per Recipe: 3
FSP: 4
Cooking Time: 20 minutes

Ingredients:
- ½ cup shredded part skim mozzarella
- Pepper and salt to taste
- ¼ cup skim milk
- 6 egg whites
- 6 eggs
- 1 zucchini, diced
- 6 pieces turkey bacon, chopped

Directions:
1. With cooking spray, lightly grease muffin tin and preheat oven to 375°F.
2. Place a nonstick cooking pan on medium fire and lightly grease with cooking spray.
3. Add bacon to pan and sauté until crisped, around 6 minutes. Transfer bacon to a plate and discard bacon fat.
4. Add zucchini to pan and sauté until tender, around 5 minutes. Transfer to plate of bacon.
5. In a large bowl, whisk egg whites and eggs. Season with pepper and salt.
6. Stir in milk, cheese, cooked zucchini, and browned bacon.
7. Evenly divide into 6 muffin tins.
8. Pop in the oven and bake for 20 minutes.
9. Serve and enjoy.

CINNAMON-APPLE OATS

Servings Per Recipe: 4
FSP: 4
Cooking Time: 15 minutes

Ingredients:
- 1/8 tsp salt
- 1 tsp cinnamon
- 1 tsp organic pure vanilla extract
- 2 tbsps honey
- 1 cup 1% organic milk
- 2 cups water
- 1 organic gala apple, peeled and diced
- ½ cup steel cut oats

Directions:
1. On medium high fire, place a medium saucepan and bring vanilla, honey, milk, and water to a boil.
2. Once boiling, quickly add oatmeal and apples and mix well. Lower fire to a simmer and cook for 10 minutes.
3. Continuously stir the mixture to prevent scorching.
4. Stir in salt and cinnamon and cook for a minute.
5. Serve and enjoy.

CHEESY, TWISTY HAM BREAD

Servings Per Recipe: 12

FSP: 3

Cooking Time: minutes

Ingredients:
- ¾ cup shredded 2% sharp cheddar cheese
- 4 tsps mustard
- 6-oz deli ham
- 1 11-oz can of Pillsbury French Bread Crusty French Loaf dough

Directions:
1. Lightly grease a baking sheet with cooking spray and preheat oven to 350°F.
2. Unroll dough to a flat rectangle. With a rolling pin, roll dough to an 11x15 rectangle. The cut the dough, in half lengthwise creating two pieces of 5.5x15-inch length dough.
3. On piece of dough, evenly spread the ham. Top with mustard and spread evenly. Then evenly spread cheese on top of mustard. Cover with the other dough and press edges with fingers to firmly seal sides.
4. With a pizza cutter, slice equally in 12 strips.
5. To twist the dough, hold one end of a strip and then twist the other side to desired number of twists. Place on prepared baking dish. Repeat process to remaining strips.
6. Pop in the oven and bake until dough is a golden brown, around 25 to 28 minutes.

Tomato and Fresh Herb Frittata

Servings Per Recipe: 4

FSP: 7

Cooking Time: 20 minutes

Ingredients:

- 1/2cup crumpled goat cheese
- 1 cup cherry tomatoes, halved
- 1 tbsp fresh parsley, chopped
- 2 tbsps basil, chopped
- 2 tbsps chives, chopped
- ¼ tsp freshly ground pepper
- ½ tsp salt
- ¼ cup 1% milk
- 8 large eggs

Directions:

1. Lightly grease a 9-inch round baking dish and preheat oven to 450of.
2. In a large bowl, whisk well pepper, salt, milk, and eggs.
3. In prepared dish, evenly spread herbs and tomatoes. Sprinkle cheese on top.
4. Pour egg mixture in baking dish.
5. Pop in the oven and bake for 20 minutes or until tops are set.
6. Evenly divide into 4, serve, and enjoy.

CHICKEN STUFFED PEPPERS

Servings Per Recipe: 4

FSP: 3

Cooking Time: 35 minutes

Ingredients:
- 4 tbsps shredded asiago cheese
- ¼ cup light ranch dressing
- 12-oz cooked, shredded chicken
- 1 tsp oil
- 1 red onion
- 4 large bell peppers of choice with tops cut and discarded, inside is hollowed out

Directions:
1. Preheat oven to 375oF.
2. On a baking dish, place peppers and bake for ten minutes to soften them.
3. Meanwhile, place a nonstick skillet on medium-high fire. Sauté onion for 8 minutes, until soft.
4. In a bowl, mix well ranch dressing, sautéed onions, and shredded chicken.
5. Once peppers are done baking, evenly stuff with the chicken mixture and return to oven
6. Bake for 30 minutes.
7. When time is up, remove peppers, sprinkle cheese on top, and return to oven. Broil for 3 minutes.
8. Then serve and enjoy.

GRAVY AND BISCUIT BAKE

Servings Per Recipe: 6
FSP: 7
Cooking Time: 30 minutes

Ingredients:
- 8-oz Jennie-O Lean Turkey Breakfast Sausage
- 1 pkg McCormick Country Gravy Mix, prepared with water
- 1 ½ cups egg beaters
- 1.75-oz can Pillsbury Buttermilk Biscuits
- 1 cup reduced fat mild cheddar

Directions:
1. Lightly grease a 9x13 baking dish with cooking spray and preheat oven to 350oF.
2. Place a nonstick skillet on medium-high fire and sauté turkey sausage until cooked, around 8 minutes. Discard fat and set aside.
3. Mix and cook the gravy mix according to package instructions.
4. Evenly spread the biscuits in bottom of baking dish.
5. Pour egg beaters on top and evenly spread sausage.
6. Pop in the oven and bake for 20 minutes.
7. Remove dish from oven and evenly sprinkle with cheese and return to oven.
8. Continue baking for another ten minutes.
9. Remove from oven, let it sit for 5 minutes before serving.

EGG SALAD SANDWICH

Servings Per Recipe: 5
FSP: 3
Prep Time: 5 minutes

Ingredients:

- 10 slices light bread, toasted if desired
- 1 tsp sugar
- 1 tbsp mustard
- 2 tbsps tartar sauce
- 6 hard-boiled eggs

Directions:

1. In a medium bowl, mash hardboiled eggs with two forks.
2. Stir in sugar, mustard, and tartar sauce. Mix well.
3. On a piece of bread, spread ¼ cup of egg mixture, and then top with another slice of bread. Repeat process to remaining egg mixture and bread slices.
4. Serve and enjoy.

EGG MUFFIN WITH BROCCOLI-CHEDDAR

Servings Per Recipe: 6

FSP: 4

Cooking Time: 15 minutes

Ingredients:

- 2 green onions, chopped
- ¾ cup reduced fat shredded cheddar cheese
- 2 cups broccoli, steamed and chopped
- Pepper and salt to taste
- ½ tbsp Dijon mustard
- 4 egg whites
- 8 eggs

Directions:

1. Lightly grease muffin tins with cooking spray and preheat oven to 350°F.
2. In a bowl, whisk well pepper, salt, mustard, egg whites, and eggs.
3. Add cheddar cheese, green onions, and broccoli.
4. Evenly divide the mixture into 12 muffin tins.
5. Pop in the oven and bake for 13 minutes or until puffy and center is set.
6. Serve and enjoy.

Egg Muffins with Black Beans

Servings Per Recipe: 6
FSP: 3
Cooking Time: 20 minutes

Ingredients:
- Pepper and salt to taste
- 4 large egg whites
- 4 large eggs
- ½ cup red onion, diced
- 1 jalapeno, seeded and diced
- 1 green bell pepper, diced
- 1 ½ cups canned black beans, rinsed and drained

Directions:
1. Lightly grease muffin tins with cooking spray and preheat oven to 350oF.
2. Place a nonstick fry pan on medium high fire and grease lightly with cooking spray. Once hot, sauté jalapeno, onion, and bell pepper for 7 minutes.
3. In a bowl, whisk well egg whites and eggs. Season with pepper and salt.
4. Once the onion mixture is done cooking, evenly divide in the 12 muffin tin.
5. Pour egg mixture on top of onion mixture.
6. Pop in the oven and bake for 23 minutes or until cooked through.
7. Serve and enjoy.

Easy Egg in a Mug with Basil and Parmesan

Servings Per Recipe: 1

FSP: 4

Cooking Time: 2 minutes

Ingredients:
- Pepper and salt to taste
- 1 tbsp Parmesan cheese
- 1 tbsp basil
- ½ cup diced tomato
- 2 egg whites
- 1 egg

Directions:
1. Lightly grease a microwave safe mug with cooking spray.
2. In mug, beat egg whites and egg. Season with salt and pepper.
3. Stir in cheese, basil, and tomato.
4. Pop in the microwave and cook for 2 minutes.
5. If egg is not set, cook for another minute.
6. Serve and enjoy.

CINNAMON-APPLE FRENCH TOAST

Servings Per Recipe: 4

FSP: 4

Cooking Time: 45 minutes

Ingredients:
- 1 cup 1% milk
- 1 1/3 cup liquid egg whites
- 4 eggs
- 2 tsps cinnamon
- 2 apples, peeled and diced
- 8 slices low calorie bread

Directions:
1. Lightly grease a 9x13-inch casserole dish with cooking spray and preheat oven to 350°F.
2. In a microwave safe bowl, mix a tsp of cinnamon with diced apples and microwave for 3 minutes.
3. In prepared casserole dish, place bread slices and evenly top with cooked apples.
4. In a bowl, whisk well milk, egg whites, and eggs. Pour over bread in casserole dish.
5. Pop in the oven and cook for 45 minutes.
6. You can serve with 2 tbsps E.D. Smith no sugar added syrup which will be an additional 1FSP.

Zucchini and Corn Frittata

Servings Per Recipe: 6

FSP: 2

Cooking Time: minutes

Ingredients:

- 2-oz sharp cheddar cheese, shredded
- ¼ tbsp dried chives
- ¼ tsp black pepper
- ¾ tsp salt
- 1/3 cup 2% plain Greek yogurt
- 8 large eggs
- 1 cup thin sliced zucchini
- 1 tbsp light butter
- 1 medium ear of fresh corn

Directions:

1. Shuck the corn and place in a bowl.
2. Lightly grease with cooking spray an oven-proof skillet and preheat oven to 350°F.
3. Place skillet on medium high fire and melt butter.
4. Sauté zucchini and corn kernels for 8 minutes. Season with pepper and salt,
5. Meanwhile, in a large bowl, whisk well eggs. Stir in cheese, basil, chives, black pepper, salt, and yogurt. Mix well.
6. Once corn and zucchini are done cooking, pour them into bowl of egg mixture and mix well.
7. Then pour egg mixture back into oven-proof skillet and lower fire to medium and let it cook for 7 minutes. Transfer skillet to oven and continue cooking for 16 minutes.
8. Turn off oven and let frittata continue cooking for another 5 minutes.

9. Remove from oven, serve and enjoy.

BAKED VEGGIE-EGG ITALIAN STYLE IN RAMEKINS

Servings Per Recipe: 4

FSP: 5

Cooking Time: 60 minutes

Ingredients:
- ¼ cup grated fat-free parmesan cheese
- 4 large eggs
- ¼ tsp black pepper
- ½ tsp salt
- ½ tsp dried basil
- 2 large garlic cloves, minced
- 1 onion, halved lengthwise, sliced
- 1 zucchini, quartered lengthwise and cut crosswise into ¾-inch chunks
- 1-lb plum tomatoes, cut into 1-inch chunks

Directions:
1. Lightly grease a shallow roasting pan and preheat oven to 400°F.
2. Place onion, zucchini, bell pepper, and tomatoes in pan. Season with pepper, salt, basil, and garlic. Toss well to coat. Pop in the oven and roast for 30 minutes or until veggies are tender.
3. After roasting, lightly grease 4 ramekins or single-serve oven proof bowls with cooking spray.
4. Evenly divide roasted vegetables in the 4 bowls and make a well in the middle.
5. Break an egg in the middle of the veggies and repeat for remaining ramekins.
6. Evenly sprinkle with cheese and bake for 23 minutes or until eggs are just set.
7. Serve and enjoy.

WEIGHT WATCHERS FREESTYLE PROGRAM LUNCH RECIPES

GRILLED TURKEY KEBABS

Servings Per Recipe:4

FSP:0

Cooking Time: 10 minutes

Ingredients:

- 1 ½ pounds lean ground turkey
- 1 egg, beaten
- ½ cup minced onion
- 2 cloves of garlic, minced
- ¼ cup fresh parsley, chopped
- ½ tsp cumin
- ½ tsp garlic powder
- ½ tsp paprika
- ¼ tsp coriander
- Salt and pepper to taste

Directions:

1. Place all Ingredients: in a large mixing bowl until well combined.
2. Press the meat mixture around wooden skewers to form kebabs. Allow to set in the fridge for 30 minutes.
3. Heat the grill to high.
4. Grill the turkey kebabs for 5 minutes on each side.

Hawaiian Chicken Kebab

Servings Per Recipe: 8

FSP:1

Cooking Time: 12 minutes

Ingredients:

- 1-pound skinless chicken breasts, cut into 2-inch chunks
- ½ cup orange juice, freshly squeezed
- ¼ cup soy sauce
- 1 tsp garlic powder
- 1 tsp onion powder
- 1 tsp black pepper
- 1 tsp salt
- ½ tsp ginger
- ½ yellow bell pepper, seeded and cubed
- ½ red bell pepper, seeded and cubed
- ½ red onion, cut into wedges
- 1 ½ cups sliced pineapple, raw

Directions:

1. In a mixing bowl, combine the chicken in orange juice, soy sauce, garlic powder, onion powder, black pepper, salt and ginger. Marinate for 2 hours inside the fridge.
2. Slide the bell pepper, onions, and pineapple, and chicken onto the skewers alternating the meat and vegetables.
3. Heat the grill to high and cook over medium flame for 6 minutes on each side or until the meat is cooked through.

CILANTRO LIME CHICKEN KABOBS

Servings Per Recipe: 8

FSP: 2

Cooking Time: 10 minutes

Ingredients:
- ¼ cup cilantro, chopped
- 2 lime fruit, juiced
- 2 tbsps olive oil
- 2 cloves of garlic, minced
- 1 tsp salt
- ½ tsp cumin
- ½ tsp paprika
- ½ tsp black pepper
- 1 ½ pounds skinless and boneless chicken breasts, chopped roughly
- 1 onion, cubed
- 2 bell peppers, cubed

Directions:
1. Place the cilantro, lime juice, olive oil, garlic, salt, cumin, paprika, and black pepper in a food processor. Pulse until smooth.
2. Place in a mixing bowl and Add the chicken breasts. Allow to marinate for 2 hours in the fridge.
3. Thread the chicken, onion, and bell peppers into skewers.
4. Heat the grill to medium and cook for 5 minutes on each side.

POTATO-CRUSTED BUTTER AND HERB TILAPIA

Servings Per Recipe: 4

FSP: 3

Cooking Time: 12 minutes

Ingredients:

- 3 tbsps light mayonnaise
- ½ tsp pickle relish
- ½ tsp lemon juice, freshly squeezed
- ½ tsp ground mustard
- 2 tbsps green onions, chopped
- 4 3-ounce tilapia fillet
- ½ cup potato flakes, organic
- Salt and pepper to taste
- ½ cup butter, melted

Directions:

1. Preheat the oven to 450^0F.
2. In a mixing bowl, combine the mayonnaise, pickle relish, lemon juice, mustard, and green onions.
3. Coat the tilapia fish with the mayonnaise mixture and then dredge on the potato flakes.
4. Press the potato flakes into the tilapia and sprinkle with salt and pepper to taste.
5. Place on a baking sheet and bake for 12 minutes.
6. Halfway through the cooking time, brush with butter.

ONE-PAN LEMON GARLIC CHICKEN AND ASPARAGUS

Servings Per Recipe: 4

FSP: 2

Cooking Time: 19 minutes

Ingredients:

- 2 tbsps flour
- 1 tsp garlic powder
- ½ tsp pepper
- ½ tsp salt
- 1 lemon, zest and juice
- 1 ½ pounds skinless chicken breast tenderloins, bones removed
- 1 tbsp olive oil
- 2 cups asparagus, chopped
- 2 cloves of garlic, minced
- ½ cup chicken broth, low sodium
- 1 tbsp white wine vinegar

Directions:

1. In a mixing bowl, combine the flour, garlic powder, pepper, salt, and lemon zest. Toss the chicken until all pieces are coated with the flour mixture.
2. Heat skillet over medium high heat and pour oil,
3. Add the coated chicken and cook on each side for 3 minutes until lightly golden.
4. Add the asparagus and garlic and cook for 3 minutes.
5. Add the chicken broth, white wine vinegar, and lemon juice. Season with more salt and pepper.
6. Close the id and simmer for 10 minutes on low heat.

BLACKENED ZUCCHINI WRAPPED FISH

Servings Per Recipe:4

FSP: 0

Cooking Time: 12 minutes

Ingredients:
- 24-ounce cod fillets, skin removed
- 1 tbsp blackening spices
- 2 zucchinis, sliced lengthwise to form a ribbon
- ½ tbsp olive oil

Directions:
1. Season the fish with the blackening spice.
2. Wrap each fish in the zucchini ribbons. Carefully place the fish on a plate
3. Heat a skillet over medium flame and pour oil.
4. Place the fish placing the sides with the ends of the zucchini ribbons down first.
5. Cook for 4 minutes on each side.

SALSA VERDE TURKEY TACOS

Servings Per Recipe: 4

FSP: 1

Cooking Time: 15 minutes

Ingredients:

- 2 tsps olive oil
- ½ onion, diced
- 2 cloves of garlic, minced
- 1 ½ pounds lean ground turkey (skinless)
- 1 tsp cumin
- ½ tsp salt
- ½ tsp pepper
- 2/3 cup salsa verde

Directions:

1. Heat the olive oil in a skillet over medium flame.
2. Sauté the onion and garlic until fragrant.
3. Stir in the lean ground turkey and season with cumin, salt and pepper.
4. Cook for 7 minutes while stirring constantly. Break the turkey meat as you go.
5. Add the salsa verde and close the lid. Allow to simmer for 5 minutes.

Easy Baked Tilapia

Servings Per Recipe: 4

FSP:2

Cooking Time: 12 minutes

Ingredients:
- ½ cup Italian breadcrumbs
- ¼ cup parmesan cheese
- 1-pound tilapia filets, rinsed and patted dry

Directions:
1. Preheat the oven to 425^0F.
2. In a bowl, combine the breadcrumbs and parmesan cheese.
3. Dredge the tilapia fillets in the breadcrumb mixture.
4. Place the coated fillets on a cooking sheet.
5. Bake for 12 minutes.

SHEET PAN HEALTHY CHICKEN PARMESAN

Servings Per Recipe: 4

FSP: 5

Cooking Time: 20 minutes

Ingredients:
- ¼ cup panko bread crumbs
- ¼ cup grated parmesan cheese
- 1 tsp garlic powder
- 1 tsp Italian seasoning
- Salt and pepper to taste
- 1-pound boneless chicken cutlets, skins removed
- 1 egg, whisked
- 3 cups green beans
- 2 tsps olive oil
- ½ cup marinara sauce, organic
- ½ cup fresh mozzarella cheese
- ¼ cup fresh basil, chopped

Directions:
1. Preheat the oven to 425°F.
2. In a mixing bowl, combine the panko breadcrumbs, parmesan cheese, garlic powder, Italian seasoning, salt, and pepper.
3. Soak the chicken breasts into the egg and dredge onto the breadcrumb mixture.
4. Place on a baking sheet. Spray with cooking oil if desired.
5. Toss the beans in olive oil and spread on the baking sheet with the chicken.
6. Cook for 15 minutes or until the chicken is cooked through.

7. Remove from the oven and pour the marinara sauce and mozzarella cheese.
8. Return to the oven and cook for 5 minutes or until the cheese melts.
9. Top with fresh basil.

Slow Chicken Cacciatore

Servings Per Recipe: 8
FSP: 0
Cooking Time: 4 hours and 5 minutes

Ingredients:

- 8 bone-in and skinless chicken thighs
- ¾ tsp salt
- A dash of ground black pepper
- 5 cloves of garlic, minced
- ½ large onion, chopped
- 1 can crushed tomatoes
- ½ medium red bell pepper, chopped
- ½ medium green bell pepper, chopped
- 4 ounces shiitake mushrooms, sliced
- 1 sprig of fresh thyme
- 1 sprig fresh oregano
- 1 bay leaf
- 1 tsp chopped parsley
- Freshly grated parmesan cheese, for serving

Directions:

1. Season the chicken with salt and pepper to taste.
2. Heat a non-stick skillet over medium heat and add the chicken. Brown for 3 minutes per side.
3. Add the garlic and onions and stir until fragrant.
4. Transfer the chicken, onion, and garlic in a slow cooker.

5. Add tomatoes, bell peppers, mushrooms, thyme, oregano, and bay leaf.
6. Season with more salt and pepper to taste.
7. Cover and cook on high for 4 hours or low for 8 hours.
8. Halfway through the cooking time, take the bay leaf out and Add parsley and cheese.

CHICKEN BURRITO BOWLS

Servings Per Recipe: 4

FSP: 6

Cooking Time: 30 minutes

Ingredients:

- 2 tsp chili powder
- 1 tsp cumin
- 1 tsp garlic powder
- ½ tsp paprika
- ¼ tsp black pepper
- ¼ tsp salt
- 1 tbsp olive oil
- 1 pound boneless and skinless chicken breasts, sliced
- 1 green pepper, sliced
- 1 red pepper, sliced
- ½ onion, sliced
- 2 cups tomatoes, chopped
- 1 can black beans, rinsed and drained
- 1 cup white rice
- 1 ½ cups chicken broth

Directions:

1. In a mixing bowl, combine the chili powder, cumin, garlic powder, oregano, paprika, black pepper, and salt. This will be the spice mixture.
2. Heat oil in a skillet over medium high heat. Stir in the chicken and half of the spice mixture. Stir constantly for 5 minutes until the chicken has turned brown.
3. Add the rest of the Ingredients: and season with the remaining spice mixture.

4. Stir to combine everything.
5. Close the lid and allow to simmer on medium flame for 25 minutes or until the rice is cooked through.

SWEET AND SOUR MEATBALLS

Servings Per Recipe: 6

FSP:1

Cooking Time: 20 minutes

Ingredients:

- 1-pound ground skinless turkey breasts
- ½ tsp salt
- 1 tsp black pepper
- 1 tsp onion powder
- 1 tsp garlic powder
- 1 tsp paprika
- 1 tsp cumin
- ¼ cup teriyaki sauce
- ¼ cup BBQ sauce, sugar-free
- 1/3 cup apple cider vinegar
- 1 tbsp brown sugar

Directions:

1. In a mixing bowl, mix together the first 7 ingredients. Mix until well-combined.
2. In another bowl, mix the remaining Ingredients: to create the sauce.
3. Roll the meat mixture into 12 small balls.
4. Place the meatballs in a baking sheet lined with parchment paper.
5. Place inside a 375°F preheated oven and bake for 10 minutes.
6. Turn the meatballs and cook for an additional 10 minutes.
7. Remove from the oven and toss in a bowl with the sauce.

ONE PAN SHRIMP FAJITAS

Servings Per Recipe: 4

FSP: 1

Cooking Time: 8 minutes

Ingredients:
- 1 tsp chili powder
- ½ tsp paprika
- ½ tsp cumin
- ½ tsp garlic powder
- ¼ tsp oregano
- ¼ tsp salt
- ¼ tsp black pepper
- 1 ½ pounds shrimps, shelled and deveined
- 2 bell peppers, sliced thinly
- 1 onion, sliced thinly
- 1 jalapeno pepper, sliced
- 2 cloves of garlic, minced
- 1 tbsp olive oil

Directions:
1. Preheat the oven to 450°F.
2. In a mixing bowl, mix together the chili powder, paprika, cumin, garlic powder, and oregano. Season with salt and pepper to taste. This will be the fajita seasoning.
3. Place the rest of the Ingredients: in a large mixing bowl and toss in the fajita seasoning.
4. Toss to coat.

5. Place on a baking sheet and spread out the shrimps.
6. Bake for 8 minutes.
7. Turn the shrimps halfway during the cooking time.

Spaghetti Squash with Shrimps and Asparagus

Servings Per Recipe: 4

FSP: 1

Cooking Time: 15 minutes

Ingredients:

- 1 spaghetti squash, large and seeded
- 1-pound asparagus, chopped
- 1 tsp olive oil
- 3 cloves of garlic, minced
- ½ cup onion, diced
- ¼ cup chicken broth, low sodium
- 1-pound shrimp, cooked and shelled
- A dash of red pepper flakes
- 1 tbsp parsley, chopped
- Salt and pepper to taste
- 2 tbsp parmesan cheese

Directions:

1. Cook the spaghetti squash in the microwave for 7 minutes. Use a fork and scrape the squash in a bowl.
2. Place the asparagus in a microwave and cook for 3 minutes. Set aside.
3. Heat the oil in a skillet over medium flame. Stir in the garlic and onions and sauté for 2 minutes. Remove from the pan and place beside the asparagus.
4. Place the broth in the skillet and allow to simmer.
5. Add the shrimps, red pepper flakes, and parsley. Season with salt and pepper to taste.

6. Assemble by placing the squash in a plate and topping it with asparagus and sautéed garlic and onions.
7. Pour in the sauce and sprinkle with parmesan cheese.

Garlic Bacon and Cheese Stuffed Chicken Breasts

Servings Per Recipe:4

FSP:4

Cooking Time: 35 minutes

Ingredients:

- 6 ounces skinless chicken breasts
- 1 egg, beaten
- 2 tbsps egg whites
- 2 ½ pounds bread crumbs
- 1 ½ tbsps parmesan cheese, grated
- 2 tbsps flour
- 1 ½ tsps garlic powder
- 1 tsp Italian seasoning
- 4-ounce light cream cheese, softened
- 3 slices of bacon, cooked and crumbled
- 1-ounce light mozzarella cheese, shredded

Directions:

1. Preheat the oven to 375^{0}F.
2. Cut the chicken breasts open until it resembles a butterfly.
3. Mix together the egg and egg whites in a bowl. Set aside.
4. In another bowl, combine the bread crumbs, parmesan cheese, flour, garlic powder, and Italian seasoning.
5. In another bowl, combine the cream cheese, and mozzarella cheese. This will be the filling.
6. Place a tbsp of the cheese mixture into the middle of the chicken breasts. Place the flaps of meat over to close over the mixture. Secure with toothpicks.

7. Submerge the chicken in the egg mixture and dredge into the bread crumbs mixture.
8. Place on a baking sheet.
9. Spray with cooking spray.
10. Bake for 35 minutes until golden brown.

MAPLE MUSTARD SALMON

Servings Per Recipe:4

FSP: 1

Cooking Time: 15 minutes

Ingredients:
- 1 ½ pounds raw wild salmon
- 3 tbsps whole grain mustard
- 2 tbsp maple syrup
- Salt and pepper to taste

Directions:
1. Preheat the oven to 350⁰F.
2. In a mixing bowl, combine all Ingredients: and make sure that the salmon is coated with the flavoring.
3. Place in a baking sheet lined with foil.
4. Bake for 15 minutes.

Turkey Apple Burgers

Servings Per Recipe: 4

FSP:1

Cooking Time: 10 minutes

Ingredients:

- 1 green apple, cored and grated
- 1-pound lean skinless ground turkey
- 1 tbsp sage, minced
- 2 tsps Dijon mustard
- ½ tsp salt
- ¼ tsp pepper
- ¼ tsp garlic powder
- ¼ tsp onion powder
- 2 tsps olive oil

Directions:

1. Mix all Ingredients: in a bowl except for the olive oil.
2. Form 4 patties using your hands.
3. Allow the patties to set on the fridge for 30 minutes prior to cooking.
4. Heat oil in a skillet over medium flame.
5. Place the turkey patties and cook on each side for 5 minutes.

SLOW COOKER TOMATO BALSAMIC CHICKEN

Servings Per Recipe: 6

FSP: 0

Cooking Time: 4 hours and 30 minutes

Ingredients:

- 2 pounds boneless and skinless chicken breasts
- 2 cups tomatoes, diced
- 1 onion, sliced thinly
- 4 cloves of garlic, minced
- 3 tbsps balsamic vinegar
- 1 tbsp Italian seasoning
- 6 cups fresh spinach
- Salt and pepper to taste

Directions:

1. Place all Ingredients: in the slow cooker except for the spinach.
2. Close the lid and cook on low for 4 hours.
3. After 4 hours, stir in the spinach and cook for 30 more minutes on high.

BLACKENED SALMON WITH GARLIC ZUCCHINI NOODLES

Servings Per Recipe: 4

FSP: 2

Cooking Time: 13 minutes

Ingredients:

- 2 tsps smoked paprika
- ½ tsp salt
- ½ tsp garlic powder
- ¼ tsp pepper
- ¼ tsp dried oregano
- 1/8 tsp chili powder
- 1 ½ pounds wild salmon fillets, skin removed
- 2 tbsps olive oil
- 2 cloves of garlic, minced
- 2 zucchinis, cut into long strips
- 1 cup cherry tomatoes
- 1 lemon, cut into wedges

Directions:

1. Create the spice rub by mixing the first 6 Ingredients: in a bowl.
2. Rub the mixture onto the salmon fillets.
3. Heat half of the oil in a skillet over medium flame and cook the salmon for 4 minutes per side. Set aside.
4. Add the remaining oil and sauté the garlic until fragrant.
5. Stir in the zucchini and tomatoes and cook for another 5 minutes.
6. Serve the vegetables with the salmon and add lemon wedges on top.

Easy Turkey Chili

Servings Per Recipe: 4

FSP:1

Cooking Time: 30 minutes

Ingredients:

- ½ tbsp olive oil
- 1 onion, chopped
- 2 cloves of garlic, minced
- 1 red pepper, chopped
- ½ cup celery, chopped
- 1 jalapeno pepper, seeded and diced
- 2 tbsps chipotle pepper, diced
- 1-pound lean ground turkey meat
- 1 ½ tbsps chili powder
- 1 tsp oregano
- 1 tsp ground cumin
- 1 bay leaf
- 1 cup tomatoes, diced
- ¾ cup chicken broth, low sodium
- Salt and pepper to taste
- 1 can kidney beans, rinsed and drained

Directions:

1. Heat oil in a skillet over medium flame.
2. Sauté the onion, garlic, red pepper, celery, jalapeno, and chipotle. Stir constantly for 5 minutes.

3. Stir in the turkey, chili powder, oregano, and ground cumin and cook for another 5 minutes.
4. Add the rest of the ingredients.
5. Allow to simmer for 20 minutes.

CREAMY CHICKEN BUBBLE UP

Servings Per Recipe: 6

FSP: 5

Cooking Time: 30 minutes

Ingredients:

- 1 8-ounce package biscuits
- 4 ounce softened light cream cheese
- 2 cups cooked shredded chicken
- 1/3 cup light sour cream
- ¼ cup ranch dressing
- 5 slices bacon, cooked and crumbled
- ½ cup low-fat cheese, shredded

Directions:

1. Preheat the oven to 375^0F.
2. Great a 9x13 baking pan with cooking spray.
3. Cut the biscuits and spread across the bottom of the baking pan.
4. In a bowl, mix together the cream cheese, sour cream, ranch dressing and chicken.
5. Spoon over the biscuits and spread evenly.
6. Bake in the oven for 30 minutes.

SLOW COOKED SKINNY SLOPPY JOES

Servings Per Recipe:

FSP: 1

Cooking Time: 6 hours

Ingredients:

- 1-pound lean ground turkey breasts
- 1 green bell pepper, chopped
- 1 onion, chopped
- ½ tsp garlic powder
- 1 can pinto beans, rinsed and drained
- 1 can tomato sauce
- 2 tsps prepared mustard1 tbsp honey
- ¼ cup sugar-free ketchup

Directions:

1. Combine all Ingredients: in a slow cooker. Stir to combine.
2. Close the lid and cook on low for 6 hours.
3. Serve with buns.

Sesame Chicken

Servings Per Recipe:6

FSP:2

Cooking Time: 30 minutes

Ingredients:

- 1 ½ tbsps sesame oil
- 1 clove of garlic, minced
- 1-pound skinless chicken breasts, cut into strips
- 2 tbsps soy sauce
- 2 tsps ground ginger
- 1 tbsp water
- 2 tbsps brown sugar
- 2 tbsps rice vinegar
- Salt and pepper to taste
- 3 tbsps sesame seeds

Directions:

1. Heat sesame oil in a skillet over medium flame.
2. Sauté the garlic until fragrant.
3. Add the chicken breast and put the rest of the Ingredients: except for the sesame seeds.
4. Close the lid and allow to cook for 15 minutes.
5. Open the lid and cook for another 5 minutes to reduce the sauce.
6. Sprinkle with sesame seeds on top.

Slow Cooked French Onion Pork

Servings Per Recipe: 4

FSP:2

Cooking Time: 8 hours

Ingredients:

- 2 ½ pounds sweet onions, sliced thinly
- 2 tbsps butter
- 2 tsps brown sugar
- 1 tbsp minced garlic
- 1 ¾ pounds boneless pork loin
- 2 packets onion soup mix

Directions:

1. Toss everything in the slow cooker.
2. Mix to combine.
3. Close the lid and cook on low for 8 hours.

WEIGHT WATCHERS FREESTYLE PROGRAM DINNER RECIPES

SLOW COOKER EASY BEEF STEW

Servings Per Recipe: 6

FSP: 3

Cooking Time: 10 hours

Ingredients:

- 1-pound skirt steak
- 1 tablespoon kitchen bouquet
- 2 tablespoons garlic salt
- 1 tablespoon black pepper
- 4 cups beef broth, low sodium
- 1-pound potatoes, cubed
- 4 medium carrots, chopped
- 3 stalks of celery, chopped

Directions:

1. Place all Ingredients: in the slow cooker.
2. Cook for 10 hours on low.
3. Once done, shred the beef and serve with the vegetables.

Chicken Marsala Meatballs

Servings Per Recipe: 10

FSP: 5

Cooking Time: 30 minutes

Ingredients:

- 8 ounces cremini mushrooms, chopped finely
- 1-pound lean ground chicken
- 1/3 cup whole wheat bread crumbs
- ¼ cup pecorino cheese, grated
- 1 large egg, beaten
- 2 tablespoons chopped parsley
- 3 cloves of garlic, minced
- 1 teaspoon salt
- A dash of black pepper
- ½ tablespoon all-purpose flour
- 1/3 cup Marsala wine
- ¾ cup chicken broth, low sodium
- ½ tablespoon unsalted butter
- ¼ cup shallots, chopped
- 3 ounces sliced shiitake mushrooms

Directions:

1. Preheat the oven to 400°F.
2. In a mixing bowl, combine the cremini mushrooms, chicken, bread crumbs, cheese, egg, parsley, garlic, salt, and pepper. Mix until well combined.
3. Form small balls using your hands and place in a greased baking sheet.
4. Bake for 20 minutes.

5. Meanwhile, make the sauce by combining the all-purpose flour, Marsala wine, and broth. Set aside.
6. Heat the butter in a skillet over medium flame and sauté the shallots until fragrant.
7. Stir in the mushrooms and cook for another 3 minutes.
8. Pour in the broth and allow to simmer for 5 minutes until it thickens.
9. Toss the cooked meatballs in to coat the sauce.

SIMPLE VEGAN POTATO SOUP

Servings Per Recipe:10

FSP: 3

Cooking Time: 35 minutes

Ingredients:

- 1 tablespoon olive oil
- 2 leeks, sliced thinly
- 1 onion, diced
- 3 cloves of garlic, minced
- 1 carrot, diced
- 2 cups potatoes, peeled and cubed
- 4 cups vegetable broth
- 2 cups water
- 2 cups rice milk
- 2 tablespoons vegan butter
- ½ cup instant potato flakes, organic
- 2 teaspoons salt
- 2 teaspoons black pepper
- 1 teaspoon onion powder
- 1 teaspoon garlic powder
- 1 teaspoon smoked paprika

Directions:

1. In a large pot, heat the oil over medium flame and sauté the leeks, onion, garlic, and carrots for 3 minutes.
2. Add the potatoes, vegetable broth, water, and rice milk. Bring to a boil.
3. Once boiled, add the rest of the Ingredients.
4. Allow to simmer for 25 minutes.

AFRICAN SWEET POTATO STEW

Servings Per Recipe: 6

FSP: 4

Cooking Time: 8 hours

Ingredients:

- 1 ¼ pounds sweet potatoes, peeled and cubed
- 2 cups diced tomatoes
- 1 can red beans, drained and rinsed
- 4 cups vegetable broth
- ½ cup water
- 1 onion, chopped
- 1 bell pepper, chopped
- 2 cloves of garlic, minced
- 1 teaspoon grated fresh ginger
- ½ teaspoon salt
- 1 teaspoon cumin powder
- ¼ teaspoon black pepper
- 3 tablespoons creamy peanut butter

Directions:

1. Place all the Ingredients: except for the peanut butter in the slow cooker.
2. Cover the lid and cook on low for 8 hours.
3. An hour before the cooking time, spoon ½ cup of the stew liquid into a bowl and dilute the peanut butter into it.
4. Stir the peanut butter mixture into the stew.
5. Close the lid and continue cooking until done.

Slow Cooker Chicken and Tomato Orzo

Servings Per Recipe: 8

FSP: 4

Cooking Time: 6 hours

Ingredients:

- 1-pound boneless chicken breasts
- 1 tablespoon olive oil
- 2 tablespoons garlic salt
- 1 tablespoon black pepper
- 2 cups chicken broth
- 8-ounce package orzo
- 2 tablespoons minced garlic
- 1 pack tomatoes, halved
- 4 tablespoons parmesan cheese, grated

Directions:

1. Place the chicken breasts, olive oil, garlic salt, pepper, and broth in a slow cooker.
2. Close the lid and cook on low for 6 hours.
3. An hour before the cooking time ends, Add the orzo, garlic, and tomatoes. Stir to combine.
4. Continue cooking
5. Serve parmesan cheese last.

Instant Pot Garlic Cuban Pork

Servings Per Recipe: 9

FSP: 5

Cooking Time: 1 hour and 20 minutes

Ingredients:

- 3 pounds boneless pork shoulder blade roast, fat removed
- 6 cloves of garlic, minced
- Juice from 1 grapefruit, freshly squeezed
- Juice of 1 lime, freshly squeezed
- ½ tablespoon fresh oregano
- ½ tablespoon cumin
- 1 tablespoon salt
- 1 bay leaf

Directions:

1. Place all Ingredients: in the Instant Pot and give a good stir.
2. Close the lid and seal the vent.
3. Adjust the cooking time to 80 minutes.
4. Do natural pressure release.
5. Remove the pork from the pressure cooker and shred using two forks.
6. Serve with tortilla, lime wedges, and salsa if desired.

CHICKEN TACO SOUP

Servings Per Recipe: 8

FSP:1

Cooking Time: 35 minutes

Ingredients:

- 1 tablespoon olive oil
- 1 onion, diced
- 1 tablespoon garlic, minced
- 1 bell pepper, diced
- 1 poblano pepper, diced
- 2 tomatoes, chopped
- 2 cups shredded chicken, cooked
- 6 cups fat-free chicken broth
- 1 cup tomato sauce
- 1 ½ cups kidney beans, rinsed and drained
- 2 tablespoons taco seasoning
- Salt and pepper to taste

Directions:

1. In a large stock pot, heat the olive oil over a medium flame. Sauté the onion and garlic until fragrant for 2 minutes.
2. Stir in the bell pepper, poblano pepper and tomatoes. Stir for 3 minutes.
3. Add the rest of the Ingredients.
4. Close the lid and allow to simmer for 30 minutes.
5. Serve with tortilla chips, cheese, and sour cream.

SHOYU AHI PORK
Servings Per Recipe:4

FSP: 0

Cooking Time: 5 minutes

Ingredients:

- 1-pound sushi grade tuna, cut into ¾-inch cubes
- ¼ cup onions, thinly sliced
- ½ cup scallions, green parts only
- 2 tablespoons reduced sodium soy sauce
- 1 teaspoon sesame oil
- ½ teaspoon sriracha or hot sauce

Directions:

1. Combine all Ingredients: in a mixing bowl.
2. Serve immediately.

GREEN CHILI CHICKEN ENCHILADA SOUP

Servings Per Recipe: 8

FSP: 3

Cooking Time: 1 hour and 10 minutes

Ingredients:

- 1-pound boneless skinless chicken breasts, roasted and shredded
- 2 cups frozen corn
- 4 cups baby spinach
- 1 white onion, diced
- 3 cloves minced roasted garlic
- 1 yellow bell pepper, diced
- 3 poblano peppers, roasted and diced
- 5 cups water
- 3 cups chicken broth, low-sodium
- 1 tablespoon cumin
- 1 tablespoon salt
- 1 teaspoon black pepper
- 1 cup fat-free sour cream

Directions:

1. In a stock pot, combine all Ingredients: except for the sour cream. Mix until well-combined. Allow to boil and simmer for 1 hour.
2. Mix in sour cream and continue cooking for 10 minutes.

Asian Chicken Soup

Servings Per Recipe: 5

FSP: 5

Cooking Time: 20 minutes

Ingredients:

- 1-pound boneless, skinless chicken breast
- 8-ounce fresh mushrooms, sliced
- 2 tablespoons lemon juice
- 1 teaspoon garlic, minced
- 1 teaspoon fresh ginger, grated
- 2 cups fat-free chicken broth
- 2 tablespoons soy sauce, reduced sodium
- 3 scallions, thinly sliced
- 1 leek, green part only

Directions:

1. Combine all Ingredients: in a pot except for the scallions and leeks.
2. Bring to a boil and allow to simmer for 15 minutes.
3. Add the scallions and leeks and continue cooking for another 5 minutes.

MEXICAN CHICKEN SOUP

Servings Per Recipe: 10

FSP: 5

Cooking Time: 6 hours

Ingredients:

- 2 cups salsa chicken, cooked and shredded
- 1 onion, chopped
- 2 cloves of garlic, minced
- 1 cup tomatoes, chopped
- 1 can great northern beans, rinsed and drained
- 1 can red kidney beans, rinsed and drained
- 1 cup whole kernel corn
- 6 cups chicken stock, fat-free
- 1 tablespoon cumin powder
- 1 teaspoon garlic powder
- 1 teaspoon onion powder
- 1 teaspoon paprika
- 1 teaspoon chili powder
- 1 teaspoon black pepper
- Salt to taste

Directions.

1. Mix all Ingredients: in a slow cooker or crockpot.
2. Cook on low heat for 6 hours.
3. Serve with tortilla chips if desired.

Easy Lentil Soup

Servings Per Recipe: 8

FSP: 0

Cooking Time: 40 minutes

Ingredients:

- 10 cups beef broth, low sodium
- 1-pound dried lentils, rinsed and drained
- 4 large carrots, chopped
- 1 large onion, chopped
- 2 celery stalks, chopped
- 2 bay leaves
- 1 ½ cups tomatoes, diced
- 1 tablespoon red wine vinegar
- Salt and pepper to taste
- 2 cups hot water

Directions:

1. In a pot, put the broth, lentils, carrots, onions, celery stalks, and bay leaves.
2. Bring to a boil and allow to simmer for 30 minutes.
3. Stir in the rest of the Ingredients.
4. Allow to simmer again for 10 more minutes.

SAUSAGE AND SPINACH SOUP

Servings Per Recipe: 4

FSP: 3

Cooking Time: 30 minutes

Ingredients:

- 10-ounce Italian turkey sausage, removed from casing
- ½ teaspoon olive oil
- 1 onion, chopped
- 4 cloves of garlic, minced
- 1 can cannellini beans
- 1 can stewed tomatoes
- 1 can chicken broth, fat-free and less-sodium
- 2 cups baby spinach
- 1 tablespoon fresh basil
- 2 teaspoons fresh oregano
- 2 tablespoons parmesan cheese, grated

Directions:

1. Place the sausages in a large saucepan and add oil. Stir until lightly golden.
2. Add the onion and garlic. Sauté for a minute or until fragrant.
3. Add the beans, tomatoes, and chicken broth. Season with salt and pepper to taste.
4. Close the lid and bring to a boil.
5. Allow to simmer for 25 minutes.
6. Add the spinach, basil, and oregano. Stir and cook for 2 more minutes.
7. Garnish with parmesan cheese on top.

SOUTHWEST GRILLED CREAM CORN

Servings Per Recipe: 8

FSP: 2

Cooking Time: 20 minutes

Ingredients:

- 16-ounce bag frozen sweet corn on the cob
- ½ cup fat-free mayonnaise
- ¼ cup grated Parmesan cheese
- ½ cup Green yogurt, plain and non-fat
- ½ teaspoon cayenne pepper
- Salt and pepper to taste

Directions:

1. Mix all Ingredients: in a bowl. Allow the corn to be coated with the rest of the Ingredients.
2. Heat the grill to medium.
3. Place the ears of corn in a cooking pan and cover with aluminum foil.
4. Place on the top shelf of the grill and cook for 20 minutes.

LENTIL AND VEGETABLE STEW

Servings Per Recipe: 6

FSP:4

Cooking Time: 8 hours and 30 minutes

Ingredients:

- 2 cups butternut squash, peeled and cubed
- 2 cups carrots, chopped
- 2 cups red potatoes, chopped
- 2 cups celery, chopped
- 1 ½ cups dry lentils, soaked overnight and rinsed
- 1 onions, diced
- 4 cloves of garlic, minced
- 8 cups vegetable broth
- 2 teaspoons herb de Provence
- 1 teaspoon salt
- 1 teaspoon smoked paprika
- 2 tablespoons olive oil
- Salt and pepper to taste
- 4 cups spinach
- ½ cup parsley

Directions:

1. Place all Ingredients: in the slow cooker except for the spinach and parsley.
2. Close the lid and cook on low for8 hours.
3. Place a blender and pulse until smooth.
4. Return to the crockpot and add the spinach and parsley.
5. Cook on high for 30 minutes.

BEEF ITALIAN SOUP

Servings Per Recipe: 8

FSP:1

Cooking Time: 30 minutes

Ingredients:

- ½ teaspoon olive oil
- ½ pound lean round steak, sliced
- ½ cup chopped onions
- 1 teaspoon Italian seasoning mix
- ¼ teaspoon garlic salt
- ¼ teaspoon pepper
- 1 can diced tomatoes, low-sodium
- ½ cup chopped carrots
- 1 can white kidney beans, rinsed and drained
- 2 cans beef broth, fat-free and low-sodium
- 2 ½ cups shredded cabbage
- ¼ cup snipped parsley

Directions:

1. Heat the oil in a pot over medium flame and stir in meat and onions. Stir for 3 minutes.
2. Season with Italian seasoning mix, garlic, salt and pepper and stir for 2 minutes.
3. Stir in the tomatoes, carrots, kidney beans and broth.
4. Bring to a boil and allow to simmer for 20 minutes.
5. Add the cabbages and parsley and allow to simmer for 5 more minutes.

GREEK LEMON CHICKEN SOUP

Servings Per Recipe: 4

FSP: 2

Cooking Time: 30 minutes

Ingredients:

- 2 cups cooked chicken, chopped
- 2 medium carrots, chopped
- ½ cup onion, chopped
- ¼ cup lemon juice
- 1 clove of garlic, minced
- 1 can cream of chicken soup, fat-free and low-sodium
- 2 cans chicken broth, fat-free
- ¼ teaspoon ground black pepper
- 2/3 cup uncooked long-grain rice
- 2 tablespoons parsley, snipped

Directions:

1. Place all Ingredients: in a pot except for the rice and parsley.
2. Season with salt and pepper to taste.
3. Bring to a boil.
4. Once the broth is boiling hot, stir in the rice.
5. Adjust the flame to medium and allow to simmer for 20 minutes until the rice is tender.
6. Garnish with parsley on top.

Turkey Vegetable Soup

Servings Per Recipe: 6

FSP: 0

Cooking Time: 23 minutes

Ingredients:

- 1 cup chopped celery
- ½ cup onion, chopped
- 1 ½ teaspoon minced garlic
- 1 ½ pounds ground turkey breasts, skinless
- 6 cups chicken broth, fat-free and low-sodium
- 1 cup carrot, sliced
- ½ cup fresh green beans, cut into 1-inch length
- ½ cup frozen whole kernel corn
- 1 ½ teaspoons ground cumin
- 1 teaspoon chili power
- 2 bay leaves
- 1 can kidney beans, rinsed and drained
- 1 can diced tomatoes and green chilies, undrained
- 6 tablespoons Monterey Jack cheese, grated

Directions:

1. Heat a non-stick pan over medium heat and add the celery, onion, garlic, and turkey. Stir for 3 minutes.
2. Add the rest of the Ingredients: except the cheese.
3. Close the lid and bring to a boil.
4. Allow to simmer for 20 minutes.
5. Serve with cheese on top.

CREAMY TOMATO BASIL SOUP

Servings Per Recipe:4

FSP: 5

Cooking Time: 15 minutes

Ingredients:

- ½ cup chopped onions
- 1 stalk celery, chopped
- 3 tablespoons olive oil
- 2 cloves of garlic, minced
- 1 cup chicken broth, fat-free and low-sodium
- 1 14-ounce can tomato puree
- Salt and pepper to taste
- 1 cup skim milk
- 5 fresh basil leaves
- 1 tablespoon cornstarch + 2 tablespoons water

Directions:

1. Place the onions and celery in a food processor and pulse until smooth.
2. Heat the oil in a pot over medium flame and pour in the onion-celery puree. Stir for 3 minutes until translucent.
3. Add the garlic, chicken broth, and tomato puree. Season with salt and pepper to taste.
4. Bring to a boil and simmer for 5 minutes.
5. Whisk in the skim milk, basil leaves, and cornstarch slurry.
6. Allow to simmer for another 5 minutes.

Unstuffed Cabbage Rolls Soup

Servings Per Recipe: 10

FSP:1

Cooking Time: 25 minutes

Ingredients:

- 1 tablespoon olive oil
- 1-pound skinless ground turkey breasts
- 1 tablespoon garlic powder
- 2 teaspoons onion powder
- 2 teaspoons Italian seasoning blend
- ¼ teaspoon chili powder
- 1 onion, chopped
- 1 clove of garlic, minced
- 1 12-ounce can tomato sauce
- 1 24-ounce can diced tomatoes
- 4 cups water
- Salt and pepper to taste.
- 1 head cabbage, shredded

Directions:

1. Heat the oil in a pot over medium flame. Stir in the ground turkey and season with garlic powder, onion powder, Italian seasoning and chili powder. Stir for 3 minutes.
2. Add the onion and garlic until fragrant.
3. Stir in the tomato sauce, diced tomatoes, and water. Season with salt and pepper to taste.
4. Cover the pot and bring to a boil.

5. Allow to simmer for 15 minutes.
6. Stir in the cabbages and cook for another 5 more minutes.

WHITE BEAN AND COLLARD GREEN SOUP WITH RICE

Servings Per Recipe:12

FSP:2

Cooking Time: 30 minutes

Ingredients:

- 1 teaspoon olive oil
- 2 stalks of celery, chopped
- 1 teaspoon minced garlic
- ½ onion, chopped
- 2 carrots, chopped
- 1 tablespoon smoked paprika
- 1 cup canned crushed tomatoes
- 1 15-ounce can diced tomatoes, drained and rinsed
- 3 sprigs of thyme
- 1 cup canned white beans, drained and rinsed
- 2 bay leaves
- 4 cups chicken stock, low-sodium
- 1 tablespoon salt
- ½ bag collard greens, washed and chopped
- 1 tablespoon sherry vinegar
- 3 cups cooked brown rice

Directions:

1. Heat the oil in a pot over medium flame and sauté the celery, garlic, and onions until fragrant.
2. Stir in the carrots, paprika, crushed tomatoes, diced tomatoes, thyme, white beans, and bay leaves. Stir for 2 minutes.

3. Pour in the stock and season with salt and pepper to taste.
4. Close the lid and bring to a boil.
5. Allow to simmer for 25 minutes.
6. Add the collard greens and sherry vinegar.
7. Cook for another 3 minutes.
8. Serve with brown rice.

TEX MEX STUFFED SUMMER SQUASH WITH BLACK BEANS

Servings Per Recipe: 4

FSP: 3

Cooking Time: 35 minutes

Ingredients:

- 2 summer squashes, halved and hollowed out
- 2 cups canned black beans, rinsed and drained
- 1 clove of garlic, minced
- ½ cup red bell pepper, diced
- 1 cup onion, minced
- ½ teaspoon cumin
- 1 cup enchilada sauce
- ½ cup cheddar cheese, grated

Directions:

1. Preheat the oven to 400^0F.
2. Heat a non-stick pan over medium flame and sauté the meat from the hollowed-out squash, black beans, garlic, red bell pepper, onion, and cumin. Stir for 7 minutes until translucent.
3. Stir in the enchilada sauce and continue cooking for 3 minutes.
4. Place the mixture back into the shells of the hollowed-out squash.
5. Sprinkle with grated cheese on top.
6. Place on a baking sheet.
7. Bake in the oven for 25 minutes.

STICKY BUFFALO CHICKEN TENDERS

Servings Per Recipe: 6

FSP: 5

Cooking Time: 20 minutes

Ingredients:

- 1-pound skinless chicken breasts, pounded into ½" thickness
- ¼ cup flour
- 3 eggs
- 1 cup panko bread crumbs
- ½ cup brown sugar
- 1/3 cup red hot sauce
- ½ teaspoon garlic powder
- 3 tablespoons water

Directions:

1. Preheat the 425°F.
2. Cut the chicken breasts into strips.
3. Place the chicken in a Ziploc bag and add the flour. Shake to coat.
4. Place the bread crumbs in a bowl.
5. Place the egg in another bowl.
6. Dip the floured meat into the eggs then into the breadcrumbs.
7. Place the chicken on a baking sheet and spray with cooking oil on top.
8. Bake in the oven for 20 minutes.
9. Meanwhile, make the sauce by mixing the remaining Ingredients: in a saucepan.
10. Serve the chicken tenders with the meat.

Chicken Fried Rice

Servings Per Recipe: 6

FSP:2

Cooking Time: 12 minutes

Ingredients:

- 1 teaspoon olive oil
- 4 large egg whites
- 1 onion, chopped
- 2 cloves of garlic, minced
- 12 ounces skinless chicken breasts, cut into ½" cubes
- ½ cups carrots, chopped
- ½ cup frozen green peas
- 2 cups long-grain brown rice, cooked
- 3 tablespoons soy sauce, low-sodium

Directions:

1. Coat a skillet with oil and heat over medium high flame.
2. Add the egg whites and cook until scrambled. Set aside.
3. Sauté the onions, garlic, and chicken breasts for 6 minutes until lightly brown.
4. Add the carrots and green peas. Continue cooking for another 3 minutes.
5. Stir in the rice and season with soy sauce.
6. Add the cooked egg whites and stir for 3 more minutes.

CHICKEN AND MUSHROOM SOUP

Servings Per Recipe:

FSP: 0

Cooking Time:

Ingredients:

- 1 chopped medium leek, white part only
- 2 cans chicken broth, low sodium
- 1 cup water
- ½ teaspoon dried thyme
- 8 ounces white mushrooms, sliced
- 1-pound skinless chicken breasts, cut into ½" inch pieces
- 8 ounces Brussels sprouts, halved
- Salt and pepper to taste

Directions:

1. Place all Ingredients: in a pot.
2. Give a good stir.
3. Close the lid and bring to a boil.
4. Allow to simmer for 15 minutes.

WEIGHT WATCHERS FREESTYLE PROGRAM SALAD AND SIDE RECIPES

INSTANT POT BRUSSELS SPROUTS WITH BACON AND GARLIC

Servings Per Recipe: 4

FSP:1

Cooking Time:

Ingredients:

- 4 slices center bacon, cut into ½" pieces
- 1-pound fresh Brussels Sprouts, halved
- 3 cloves of garlic, minced
- 3 shallots, chopped

Directions:

1. Turn the Instant Pot to the Sauté setting.
2. Add the bacon until crispy.
3. Stir in the rest of the Ingredients.
4. Close the lid and seal the vent.
5. Press the Manual button and adjust the cooking time to 4 minutes.
6. Do quick pressure release.

HEALTHY TUNA SALAD WRAPS

Servings Per Recipe:2

FSP:1

Cooking Time: 5 minutes

Ingredients:

- 1 12-ounce can tuna, in water and low-sodium
- 1 hard-boiled egg, sliced
- ¼ small onion, chopped
- 1 tsp dill pickle relish
- 2 tbsps Greek yogurt, plain
- 1 tsp mayonnaise
- ½ tsp garlic powder
- ½ tsp black pepper
- ¼ tsp salt
- 1 head Bibb lettuce
- ½ cup tomatoes, halved

Directions:

1. Drain the water from the tuna.
2. In a bowl, combine the tuna, eggs, onion, pickle, yogurt, mayonnaise, garlic powder, black pepper, and salt.
3. Scoop on lettuce leaves and top with tomatoes.

Caesar Salad

Servings Per Recipe: 5

FSP:2

Cooking Time: 5 minutes

Ingredients:

- 1/3 cup non-fat Greek yogurt, plain
- ¼ cup mayonnaise, reduced-fat
- 1 tbsp red wine vinegar
- 2 tsps Dijon mustard
- 1 tsp Worcestershire sauce
- 10 cups romaine lettuce, washed and drained
- 30 fresh croutons
- 2 ½ tbsps parmesan cheese, grated

Directions:

1. In a small bowl, mix the yogurt, mayonnaise, red wine vinegar, mustard, and Worcestershire sauce.
2. Shred the romaine lettuce and place in a salad bowl.
3. Top with the salad dressing and mix.
4. Garnish with croutons and parmesan cheese.

HEALTHY CHICKEN SALAD RECIPE

Servings Per Recipe: 6

FSP:1

Cooking Time: 5 minutes

Ingredients:

- 2 cups cooked chicken breasts, chopped
- ½ cup non-fat Greek yogurt
- ¼ cup non-fat sour cream
- 1 tbsp mayonnaise
- ½ gala apple chopped into small pieces
- 2 tbsps bell pepper, minced
- 1 tbsp dill pickle relish
- 1 tsp garlic powder
- 1 tsp onion powder
- ½ tsp paprika
- ½ tsp black pepper

Directions:

1. In a large bowl, mix all Ingredients: until well combined.
2. Serve with bread or crackers if desired.

Black Bean and Corn Salad

Servings Per Recipe: 4

FSP: 0

Cooking Time: 5 minutes

Ingredients:

- 1 cup canned black beans, rinsed and drained
- 1 cup corn
- 1 red pepper, chopped
- 1 cup cherry tomatoes, chopped
- ½ cup red onion, chopped
- 1 tbsp fresh lime juice
- 1 tsp ground cumin
- 1 tsp hot sauce

Directions:

1. Mix all Ingredients: in a salad bowl.
2. Season with salt and pepper to taste.
3. Refrigerate before serving.

CHICKPEA GREEK SALAD

Servings Per Recipe: 5

FSP: 4

Cooking Time: 5 minutes

Ingredients:

- 1 tbsp olive oil
- 1 tbsp red wine vinegar
- 2 tbsp lemon juice
- 2 cloves of garlic, minced
- 1 tsp oregano
- Salt and pepper to taste
- 20 ounces canned chickpeas, rinsed and drained
- 1 red pepper, chopped
- 1 green bell pepper, chopped
- 1 cup red onion, chopped
- 1 cup red onion, chopped
- 1 ½ cups cherry tomatoes, halved
- 1 cucumber, chopped
- ½ cup celery, chopped
- ¼ cup parsley, chopped
- ¼ cup feta cheese
- ½ cup Kalamata olives, chopped

Directions:

1. In a small bowl, combine the olive oil, red wine vinegar, lemon juice, garlic, oregano, salt and pepper. This will be the salad dressing.
2. In a bigger bowl, mix the rest of the Ingredients. Pour in the salad dressing.
3. Toss to combine everything.

HEALTHY SALMON PANZANELLA SALAD

Servings Per Recipe: 6

FSP: 3

Cooking Time: 5 minutes

Ingredients:

- 3 tbsps extra virgin olive oil
- 2 tbsps red wine vinegar
- ½ tsp Dijon mustard
- ½ tsp salt
- ¼ tsp pepper
- 8 ounces green beans, trimmed and steamed until tender
- 4 cups whole wheat baguette, cut into cubes
- 2 cups cherry tomatoes, halved
- 1 cup red onions, sliced thinly
- ½ cup fresh basil leaves, chopped
- 1 can wild Alaskan salmon, drained and skin removed

Directions:

1. In a small bowl, mix together the olive oil, red wine vinegar, Dijon mustard, salt and pepper
2. In a salad bowl, combine all Ingredients: and pour in the dressing.
3. Toss the salad.
4. Place in the fridge to chill before serving.

VEGAN BEST STUFFING RECIPE

Servings Per Recipe: 10

FSP: 4

Cooking Time: 20 minutes

Ingredients:

- 5 cups Pepperidge Farm Cubed Stuffing
- 3 cups fat-free vegetable broth
- ¼ cup vegan butter
- 2 tbsp dry Vegetable Soup Mix
- 2 cloves of garlic, minced
- 2 tsps onion powder
- 2 tsps dried sage
- 1 tsp dried marjoram

Directions:

1. Heat the oven to 325^{0}F.
2. In a bowl, mix all Ingredients: until well-combined.
3. Place in a casserole dish.
4. Bake for 20 minutes.

Turkey Taco Salad

Servings Per Recipe:5

FSP:2

Cooking Time: 10 minutes

Ingredients:

- 1-pound fat-free ground turkey
- 1 sweet red pepper, chopped
- 1 sweet yellow pepper, chopped
- 1/3 cup chopped onion
- 1 ½ cups salsa
- 2 tsps chili powder
- 1 tsp ground cumin
- 8 cups romaine lettuce, torn
- 10 tortilla chips
- 5 tbsps cheddar cheese, grated

Directions:

1. Heat a non-stick pan over medium flame and stir in the turkey, peppers, and onion. Keep stirring for 6 minutes until the turkey is no longer pink.
2. Stir in the salsa, chili powder, and cumin. Season with salt and pepper to taste.
3. Cook for another 4 minutes.
4. Serve on top of romaine lettuce and garnish with tortilla chips and cheddar cheese.

BLACK BEAN AND CORN SALAD WITH AVOCADO

Servings Per Recipe: 8

FSP: 2

Cooking Time: 5 minutes

Ingredients:

- 1 tsp cumin
- ¼ cup balsamic vinegar
- ½ tsp salt
- ½ tsp black pepper
- 1 can black beans, rinsed and drained
- 1 10-ounce package frozen corn
- 1 large tomato, diced
- 1 large cucumber, diced
- 1 bunch cilantro, chopped
- 1 ripe medium avocado, seeded and diced
- 1 clove of garlic, minced
- Juice from 1 lime, freshly squeezed
- 1 tbsp olive oil

Directions:

1. In a small bowl, mix cumin, balsamic vinegar, salt and pepper. Set aside.
2. In a large salad bowl, mix the beans, corn, tomato, cucumber, cilantro, avocado, and garlic.
3. Pour in lemon juice, olive oil, and balsamic vinaigrette.
4. Toss to coat the vegetables.

ITALIAN CHOPPED SALAD

Servings Per Recipe: 4

FSP: 3

Cooking Time: 5 minutes

Ingredients:

- 8 cups romaine lettuce, washed and rinsed
- 1 cup chopped tomatoes
- 1 cup rotini pasta, cooked according to package instruction
- 2 slices crispy bacon, crumbled
- 1-ounce cheddar cheese, cut into small cubes
- ¼ cup fat-free Italian dressing

Directions:

1. Mix all Ingredients: in a salad bowl.
2. Toss to coat.
3. Season with salt and pepper if needed.
4. Chill before serving.

Chicken Pot Pasta

Servings Per Recipe: 8

FSP: 5

Cooking Time: 35 minutes

Ingredients:

- 1 ½ pounds boneless and skinless chicken breasts
- 4 tbsps light butter
- ½ cup chopped onion
- ¼ cup flour
- ½ tsp salt
- ¼ tsp black pepper
- 1 ½ cups skim milk
- 2 ½ cups water
- ½ tsp poultry seasoning
- 8 ounces uncooked egg noodles
- 1 cup frozen corn kernels
- 2 cups frozen peas and carrots

Directions:

1. Place the chicken breasts in a pot and cover with water to about 2 inches over the chicken.
2. Bring to a boil on high heat then adjust the heat to medium and allow to simmer for 20 minutes.
3. Take the chicken out and chop and set aside.
4. In the pot, melt the butter over medium flame and sauté the onion for 2 minutes.
5. Whisk the flour, salt and pepper for a minute.

6. Add the milk and water. Whisk until well combined.
7. Bring to a boil and add the egg noodles, corn, and vegetables.
8. Allow to simmer for 8 minutes until the noodles are cooked.
9. Top with the chopped chicken

YOGURT-FILLED CANTALOUPE

Servings Per Recipe:1

FSP:0

Cooking Time: 5 minutes

Ingredients:

- ½ cantaloupe, seeded
- 6 ounces non-fat Greek yogurt
- 1 tbsp fresh strawberries
- 1 tbsp fresh blueberries
- 1 tsp raw pepita seeds

Directions:

1. Fill the hole of the cantaloupe with non-fat Greek yogurt.
2. Add the berries then sprinkle with pepitas.
3. Chill in the fridge before serving.

Summer Fruit Salad with Mint and Almonds

Servings Per Recipe: 4

FSP:1

Cooking Time: 5 minutes

Ingredients:

- 4 apricots, pitted and sliced
- 1 6-ounce can blueberries
- 1 6-ounce can raspberry
- 6 ounces strawberries, fresh
- Zest and juice from 1 lemon
- ½ bunch mint
- ¾ cup Marcona almonds
- 3 tbsps sugar

Directions:

1. Place all Ingredients: in a mixing bowl.
2. Toss to coat.
3. Chill inside the fridge before serving.

PEAR AND BLUE CHEESE SALAD

Servings Per Recipe: 4

FSP: 3

Cooking Time: 5 minutes

Ingredients:

- ¼ cup pear nectar
- 2 tbsps walnut oil
- 2 tbsps white wine vinegar
- 1 tsp Dijon mustard
- 1/8 tsp ground ginger
- 1/8 tsp ground black pepper
- 1 tsp honey
- 10 cups mesclun greens, torn
- 3 medium green pears, cored and sliced
- ½ cup walnuts, broken
- ½ cup crumbled blue cheese

Directions:

1. Place in a small bowl the pear nectar, walnut oil, white wine vinegar, mustard, ginger, black pepper, and honey. Whisk until well combined. Set aside.
2. In a mixing bowl, combine the mesclun greens, pears, walnuts, and blue cheese.
3. Pour over the dressing.
4. Toss to coat.
5. Chill before serving.

WEIGHT WATCHERS FREESTYLE PROGRAM SNACKS AND DESSERT RECIPES

No-Bake Blueberry Cheesecake

Servings Per Recipe: 8

FSP: 5

Prep Time: 5 minutes

Ingredients:

- 1 pint blueberries, divided
- 10 Pizelle cookies, vanilla
- ½ cup whipped cream cheese
- 1 8-oz container fat-free whipped topping
- 2 cups skim milk
- 1 sugar-free vanilla pudding mix

Directions:

1. In a casserole dish, spread cookies in a single layer.
2. Mix well for 5 minutes the skim milk and pudding mix in a large bowl, or until thickened.
3. Fold in cream cheese.
4. And spread ½ of the cream cheese mixture on top of cookies.
5. Sprinkle 1/3 of the blueberries in an even layer on top of cream cheese.
6. Pour remaining cream cheese mixture on top of blue berries and then cover top with remaining blueberries.
7. Cover and place in the fridge for at least 2 hours before serving.

Ranch Dressing and Dip in One

Servings Per Recipe: 4
FSP: 0
Prep Time: 5 minutes

Ingredients:
- ¼ tsp paprika
- ½ tsp dill weed
- 1 tsp pepper
- 1 tsp sea salt
- 1 tsp onion powder
- 1 tsp dried chives
- 1 tsp dried parsley
- 2 tbsps milk
- 1 cup non-fat plain Greek yogurt

Directions:
1. In a bowl with lid, whisk all Ingredients: until thoroughly combined.
2. Cover and place in the fridge until ready to use for up to 2 weeks.

CINNAMON-APPLE MUFFINS

Servings Per Recipe: 18

FSP: 3

Cooking Time: 18 minutes

Ingredients:
- 2 tsps ground cinnamon
- 1 cup water
- 1 small ripe banana
- ½ cup unsweetened applesauce
- 1 ½ cups Granny Smith apples, chopped
- 1 sugar-free cake mix

Directions:
1. Line 18 muffin tins with liner and preheat oven to 375°F.
2. In a large bowl, mash bananas. Pour in water and applesauce. Mix well.
3. Stir in cinnamon and cake mix. Mix well.
4. Add chopped apples and mix well.
5. Evenly pour batter in 18 muffin tins.
6. Pop in the oven and bake until tops are golden brown and cooked through, around 18 minutes.

Easy Cornbread Recipe

Servings Per Recipe: 12
FSP: 3
Cooking Time: 30 minutes

Ingredients:
- ½ tsp salt
- 1 tsp pepper
- 1 ½ cups vegetarian jiffy mix
- 1 cup fat-free plain Greek yogurt
- 1 ½ cups whole kernel corn

Directions:
1. Lightly grease and 8x8 ovenproof dish and preheat oven to 375°F.
2. Mix well yogurt, salt, and pepper.
3. Stir in jiffy mix. Mix well.
4. Add corn and mix well.
5. Spread in prepared dish and pop in the oven.
6. Cook until tops are starting to lightly brown and cooked through, around 30 minutes.

Blueberry and Lemon Protein Muffins

Servings Per Recipe: 15

FSP: 5

Cooking Time: 25 minutes

Ingredients:

- 1 ¼ cups blueberries
- 1 tsp vanilla extract
- 2 tsps pure lemon extract
- 3 tbsps lemon juice
- 1/3 cup canola oil
- ½ cup sugar
- ½ tsp salt
- 2 tsps baking soda
- 2 scoops vanilla protein powder
- 1 ½ cups white whole wheat flour
- 1 cup unsweetened soy milk
- 1 tsp apple cider vinegar

Directions:

1. Line 15 muffin tins with liner and preheat oven to 350°F.
2. In a large bowl, whisk well vanilla extract, lemon extract, lemon juice, canola oil, salt, baking soda, soy milk, and vinegar. Mix well.
3. Stir in sugar and mix well.
4. Add protein powder and mix thoroughly.
5. Stir in flour and mix well.
6. Fold in blueberries and evenly divide in prepared muffin tins.
7. Pop in the oven and bake until tops are lightly browned and cooked through, around 25 minutes.

Vegan Approved Brownies

Servings Per Recipe: 12
FSP: 1
Cooking Time: 35 minutes

Ingredients:
- ½ tsp baking powder
- ½ tsp salt
- ¼ cup all-purpose flour
- 1/3 cup unsweetened cocoa powder
- ¼ cup unsweetened applesauce
- ¼ cup blackstrap molasses
- 1 ½ cups black beans

Directions:
1. Lightly grease an 8x8 ovenproof dish with cooking spray and preheat oven to 375°F.
2. Wash black beans and drain thoroughly. Puree in blender and pour in a medium mixing bowl.
3. Mix in baking powder, salt, applesauce, and molasses. Mix well.
4. Stir in flour and cocoa powder. Mix thoroughly.
5. Pour batter in prepared dish and pop in the oven. Cook until cooked through, around 35 minutes.

BEAN DIP HOMEMADE

Servings Per Recipe: 8

FSP: 0

Cooking Time: 3 Hours

Ingredients:

- ½ cup mild salsa
- 1 tsp black pepper
- 1 tsp chili powder
- 1 tsp salt, divided
- 2 tsps cumin, divided
- 1 tsp onion powder, divided
- 1 tsp garlic powder, divided
- 2 cups water
- 1 cup dry pinto beans

Directions:

1. Add water in slow cooker. Rinse pinto beans and add to slow cooker.
2. Stir in half of the salt, cumin, onion powder, and garlic powder. For 3 hours cook beans on high.
3. Transfer beans in a sieve and drain all water. Once thoroughly drained, transfer beans to a bowl.
4. Stir in remaining spices and seasoning. Add salsa and mix well.
5. If desired, you can mash beans to desired consistency.

Coconut and Banana Muffins

Servings Per Recipe: 12

FSP: 4

Cooking Time: 17 minutes

Ingredients:

- 2 tsps baking powder
- 1 tsp salt
- ¾ cup whole wheat flour
- ¼ cup unsweetened coconut flakes
- ½ cup quick cooking oats
- 1 tsp vanilla
- 2 egg whites
- 1 cup Splenda
- ¼ cup coconut oil
- 3 ripe bananas

Directions:

1. Line a dozen muffin tin with liner and preheat oven to 375°F. Mash bananas in a large bowl.
2. Whisk in vanilla, egg whites, and coconut oil. Mix well.
3. Stir in baking powder, Splenda, and salt. Mix well.
4. Add flour, coconut flakes, and oats. Mix well.
5. Evenly divide batter into 12 muffin tins.
6. Pop in the oven and bake until tops are lightly browned, around 17 minutes.

LOADED POTATO DIP

Servings Per Recipe: 8

FSP: 1

Cooking Time: 10 minutes

Ingredients:

- 1/8 tsp onion powder
- ¼ tsp garlic powder
- 1/8 tsp salt
- 1/8 tsp black pepper
- 1 tbsp chives
- 1/8 cup shredded 2% sharp cheddar cheese
- 2 strips Turkey bacon, cooked crisp and crumbled
- 1 cup fat free sour cream

Directions:

1. In a small bowl with lid, mix all Ingredients: thoroughly.
2. Cover and refrigerate for at least an hour.
3. Serve with slices of carrots, celery, or even reduced fat chips.

COOKIES APPLE PIE FLAVORED

Servings Per Recipe: 24
FSP: 2
Cooking Time: 12 minutes

Ingredients:
- ½ tsp cinnamon
- 1 cup apple, diced
- 2 eggs
- ½ cup unsweetened applesauce
- 1 box sugar-free yellow cake mix

Directions:
1. Lightly grease 2 baking sheets with cooking spray and preheat oven to 375oF.
2. Whisk eggs in a medium bowl. And add applesauce and mix well.
3. Stir in cinnamon and cake mix. Mix well.
4. Add diced apples and mix.
5. Scoop 1-inch balls of the batter and place at least 2-inches apart in the prepared baking sheet.
6. Pop in the oven and bake to desired doneness or around 10 to 12 minutes.

Jalapeno, Bacon, and Corn-Cheese Dip

Servings Per Recipe: 10

FSP: 3

Cooking Time: 20 minutes

Ingredients:

- 2 cups shredded cheddar cheese
- ¼ cup parmesan cheese
- 8-oz cream cheese, softened
- ¼ cup diced jalapenos
- 2 cans corn, drained
- 8 strips bacon, cooked and crumbled

Directions:

1. Prepare a cast iron skillet and preheat oven to 400°F.
2. In a bowl, mix well all Ingredients.
3. Transfer Ingredients: into prepared skillet and pop in the oven.
4. Bake for 20 minutes.
5. Serve and enjoy with chips which is an additional FSP depending on variety of chips.

OAT AND BANANA PROTEIN SNACK BALLS

Servings Per Recipe:
FSP: 1
Prep Time: 10 minutes

Ingredients:

- 1 large banana
- 1 serving vanilla protein powder
- 1 cup rolled oats

Directions:

1. In a blender, add protein powder and oats. Pulse until nearly smooth.
2. Add banana to blender and continue pulsing until you make a dough.
3. Evenly divide dough into 12 balls.
4. Store in an air tight container and snack on it as desired.

DELICIOUS PUMPKIN CUPCAKES

Servings Per Recipe: 24

FSP: 2

Cooking Time: 22 minutes

Ingredients:
- 1 cup water
- 1 15-oz can 100% pumpkin puree
- 1 box sugar-free yellow cake mix

Directions:
1. Line 2 dozen muffin tins with liner and preheat oven to 350oF.
2. In a large bowl, mix well all Ingredients.
3. Evenly divide into 24 muffin tins and pop in the oven.
4. Bake for 22 minutes or until tops are lightly browned.

Oatmeal and Blueberry Muffins

Servings Per Recipe: 12
FSP: 5
Cooking Time: 24 minutes

Ingredients:
- 1 cup fresh blueberries
- ½ tsp salt
- ½ tsp baking soda
- 1 tsp baking powder
- 2/3 cup all-purpose flour
- 1 tsp vanilla extract
- 1 tbsp canola oil
- 2 large egg whites
- 1/2 cup unsweetened applesauce
- 2 tbsps honey
- ½ cup brown sugar, packed
- 1 cup unsweetened almond milk
- 1 ½ cups oats

Directions:
1. Pulse the oats in a blender until coarse and then soak in almond milk for at least 30 minutes.
2. After 30 minutes, with liner line 12 muffin tins and preheat oven to 400°F.
3. In a large bowl, whisk well salt, baking soda, baking powder, vanilla extract, canola oil, egg whites, applesauce, and honey. Mix thoroughly.
4. Stir in flour, brown sugar, and soaked oats. Mix well.

5. Evenly divide in prepared muffin tins and pop in the oven.
6. Bake until tops are browned, around 24 minutes.

LEMONY PUDDING DESSERT

Servings Per Recipe: 3
FSP: 1
Cooking Time: 10 minutes

Ingredients:
- 1 fat-free whipped topping
- 1 1/3-oz sugar-free lemon gelatin mix
- 2 cups water
- 1 7/8-oz sugar-free vanilla cook and serve pudding mix, not instant

Directions:
1. Place a saucepan on medium high fire and add water.
2. With a whisk, stir in pudding mix slowly while whisking continuously.
3. Bring to a boil and once pudding is thickened, whisk in gelatin while whisking continuously.
4. Evenly pour into three dessert dishes and place in the fridge for 2 hours or until cooled.
5. To serve, top with whipped topping.

Made in the USA
Lexington, KY
07 March 2018